Intermittent Fasting

Learn The Simple And Proven Method For Losing Weight, Reversing Chronic Disease, And Anti-Aging!

By Kris Kemp

Table of Contents

INTRODUCTION...I

CHAPTER ONE: WHAT IS AUTOPHAGY?.................................. 2

CHAPTER TWO: METHODS OF INTERMITTENT FASTING .. 8

CHAPTER THREE: HOW TO GO ABOUT INTERMITTENT
FASTING 15

CHAPTER FOUR: INTERMITTENT FASTING AND WEIGHT
LOSS 20

CHAPTER FIVE: FASTING AND HUMAN GROWTH
HORMONE 24

CHAPTER SIX: COMMON FAQS 29

CHAPTER SEVEN: FASTING AND THE KETOGENIC DIET ... 39

CHAPTER EIGHT: WHAT WORKS BEST? 45

CHAPTER NINE: FASTING AND EXERCISING...........................51

CONCLUSION...55

RESOURCES 57

Introduction

Thank you for purchasing Intermittent Fasting – Learn The Simple And Proven Method For Losing Weight, Reversing Chronic Disease, And Anti-Aging! This is your first step in a life-changing journey!

Do you want to learn about a nutritional plan that will help you attain your weight loss goals without having to reduce your daily food intake drastically? Does this sound appealing? If you want to achieve your health and fitness goals, then your perfect way to eat is intermittent fasting! Instead of fretting about *what* you eat, you need to start paying attention to *when* you eat while following this way of life.

There are many different benefits that intermittent fasting offers, and they will all be discussed thoroughly. Potentially the most significant and exciting of all the benefits is autophagy. Autophagy is a natural internal mechanism that helps regulate the process of cellular regeneration and waste removal. When autophagy functions optimally, it helps improve one's overall health and well-being.

In addition to an in-depth look at autophagy, this book will provide you with a full rundown on the different methods and advantages of intermittent fasting, FAQs about intermittent fasting, and potential concerns with this particular way of eating.

With that being said...

Read on!

Chapter One:

What is Autophagy?

Autophagy is a natural process that occurs in the body wherein the body starts to, for lack of better phrasing, eat itself slowly. That thought may sound scary initially, so it is essential to learn about this process and the benefits it offers. There is nothing unnatural or harmful about autophagy. This internal process is necessary for the body to cleanse itself internally and remove all the damaged cells and toxins to improve one's health while generating healthy cells in the body. In its normal functioning (and because of unhealthy habits), the human body tends to accumulate various dead organelles like proteins and different oxidized particles that clog up its internal mechanisms.

The buildup of all these toxins in the body makes it vulnerable to the risk of different diseases like dementia, cancer and several other disorders related to the aging of cells. Since there are millions of cells present in the human body, it is obvious that these cells need some maintenance and repair from time to time so that they function optimally. The human body has a unique internal system that helps get rid of any faulty cells and enables it to protect itself from diseases. All this means that autophagy is a natural defense mechanism and is quite essential.

Before moving onto the technical aspects of this function, here is a simple analogy that will give you a better understanding of autophagy. The human body is like a kitchen. After a meal is cooked, the kitchen must be scrubbed clean, garbage must be taken out and whatever can be recycled must be recycled. Similarly, the human body needs upkeep. The mechanism that does all the cleaning is autophagy. Now, think of a situation where you are a couple of years older and aren't as effective as you once were. After you cook a meal, you might leave stuff out on the countertop; some might be thrown away into the garbage while the rest stays on the countertop. The food might rot and give out different kinds of nasty odors. All of this will lead to a buildup of toxic waste in the kitchen. If this happens, it becomes doubly difficult to clean the kitchen. This situation is similar to what will happen in your body if autophagy doesn't do its job.

Autophagy usually works in the background as it helps with the regular maintenance of the body. Autophagy kicks in during high-stress situations to enhance the body's natural defense mechanism. In this way, autophagy helps the body resist diseases and boosts longevity. Admittedly, autophagy is a wondrous process in the human body. Perhaps even more remarkable is that it's possible to increase the body's autophagy mechanism. Information about doing so will come later in the book.

Benefits of Autophagy

Autophagy helps maintain homeostasis. What is homeostasis? It is essentially having balanced cellular function in the body. Homeostasis, as well as vibrant health, is the result of a protein called p62 working its magic during autophagy[1]. All of the damaged cells that are accumulated in the body over time are removed, and this creates space for new cells to form. This process does sound good, but what are the noticeable benefits of autophagy?

---

[1] Liu, W., Ye, L., Huang, W., Guo, L., Xu, Z., & Wu, H. et al. (2016). p62 links the autophagy pathway and the ubiqutin–proteasome system upon ubiquitinated protein degradation. *Cellular & Molecular Biology Letters*, 21(1). doi: 10.1186/s11658-016-0031-z

Change in the functioning of cells
When the human body doesn't consume food for a period of time, multiple things happen within the body. For instance, the process of cellular repair and regeneration starts. Additionally, hormone levels in the body change, making fat available for generating energy. While in a state of fasting, the body's insulin level drops, and low insulin facilitates the burning of fat. On the other hand, the level of growth hormone spikes. Still another benefit in cellular functioning is that several genes and molecules undergo positive changes in composition to improve longevity and immunity against diseases.

Losing weight and belly fat
Most people who take up intermittent fasting do it with the primary aim of losing weight. Intermittent fasting ensures that there is a restriction on food intake. Anyone will end up consuming fewer calories on this plan as long as they don't try to compensate for fasting times by overeating during the other times. Intermittent fasting also helps in enhancing the function of hormones that influence weight loss. Fat molecules break due to lower levels of insulin, a higher level of growth hormone, and noradrenaline. Most of the fat that is shed comes from the abdominal cavity. And intermittent fasting helps in improving metabolism, while also helping to cut down the calories one consumes.

Reducing insulin resistance
Intermittent fasting can have drastic impacts upon disease, including diabetes. One of the most common forms of diabetes that can be tackled with intermittent fasting is Type 2 diabetes. In this condition, the levels of blood sugar are high, and there is resistance to insulin in the body. Anything that helps to reduce resistance towards insulin helps to reduce the levels of blood sugar in the body. It has been shown that intermittent fasting helps in reducing insulin resistance in the body. A study that was conducted on diabetic rats has shown that this fasting helps in protecting them from kidney damage and the other complications that accompany diabetes.

Reducing inflammation

Oxidative stress pushes the body a step closer towards aging and chronic diseases. Oxidation occurs when unstable molecules react with useful molecules like protein or DNA and damage them in the process. Several studies show that intermittent fasting can successfully improve the body's resistance to oxidative stress.

It's good for the heart

Heart disease is one of the greatest threats to human health today. Intermittent fasting holds much promise for stemming the progress of this disease because it helps to improve various risk factors for heart disease, like blood pressure, good cholesterol, level of triglycerides, and levels of blood sugar. However, it is important to note that most of the data supporting these claims has been collected from animal studies.

Cell repair

At the start of a fast, the cells in the body begin the process of waste removal. This process involves breaking down dysfunctional cells and proteins within them (autophagy). An increase in autophagy helps in providing some additional protection against cancer and other diseases like Alzheimer's. It facilitates the removal of waste that has been building up in cells.

It can be life-saving

It might sound a tad dramatic, but it is entirely true. It is scientifically accurate. Autophagy's primary purpose is life preservation. During a time of severe stress like infection or even starvation, the process of autophagy is kickstarted and helps optimize the process of repair while reducing damage. Intermittent fasting activates autophagy, which can starve almost any infectious intruder of glucose. By doing so, inflammation is reduced, making it easier for the immune system to repair the damage that inflammation and infections cause. In short, the autophagy mechanism has evolved in such a manner that it helps save energy and repairs damage when power is scarce. It is essential for the immune system's defense mechanism to fight any illness.

May promote longevity

Anti-aging benefits may sound mythical, but beauty isn't merely skin deep – it runs deeper. Scientists discovered autophagy during the 1950s, and since then there have been several studies that were and are still being conducted to understand how autophagy improves cellular function and health. One thing that is certain is that cells don't take in additional nutrients during autophagy. Instead, they tend to replace their damaged parts, get rid of any toxic material inside, and start to fix themselves. When the cells in the body begin to repair themselves, they indeed tend to work better, and they act like younger cells. You might have noticed that some people appear to have a different chronological vs. biological age. The toxic damage that your body experiences and its ability to repair this situation plays a significant role in these differences.

Better metabolism

Autophagy is similar to a housekeeping service. Not only does it take the trash out, but it replaces vital cell parts like mitochondria. Mitochondria are the powerhouses in a cell. They burn fat and produce ATP, the body's energy currency. Autophagy helps your cells function more effectively and efficiently, and it also helps synthesize new proteins. All this makes your cells healthy and this, in turn, improves your metabolism.

Reduction in the risk of neurodegenerative diseases

Most of the conditions related to the aging of the brain take a long time to develop, since the proteins present in and around the brain cells are misfolded, and they don't function like they are supposed to. Autophagy helps clean up all these malfunctioning proteins and reduces the accumulation of such proteins. For instance, autophagy helps remove amyloid and α-synuclein in Parkinson's[2]. There is a reason why it is believed that dementia and diabetes go hand in hand with each other – the consistently high levels of blood sugar prevent autophagy from kicking in, and this makes it difficult for cells to get rid of the clutter.

Better skin health

The cells of the body are susceptible to a variety of damage from chemicals, air, light, humidity, pollution and all forms of physical harm. Given all that the body's exterior, skin, is exposed to, it's noteworthy that most people don't look worse than they do. When your skin cells start to accumulate damage and toxins, they begin to age. Autophagy helps repair and replace these cells, and it makes your skin look fresh. Skin cells also tend to engulf bacteria that can damage the body, so it is essential to support them as they are clearing the clutter. Because of this natural process of revitalization, the damaging effects of environmental conditions do not appear as drastic.

Healthy weight

Short periods of fasting help the body to activate autophagy, burn fat, hold onto muscle mass and make the body lean and fit. Fasting also reduces the chances of unnecessary inflammation that usually leads to weight gain. Autophagy helps reduce the levels of toxins in your body, and when this happens, the cells in your body will not retain as much fat. Autophagy also supports your metabolic efficiency by repairing those parts of the cells that usually create and package proteins and synthesize energy, which is helpful when the batteries need to start burning fat to provide power.

---

[2] The 12 Important Benefits Of Autophagy. (2019). Retrieved from https://www.naomiwhittel.com/the-12-important-benefits-of-autophagy/

Chapter Two:

Methods of Intermittent Fasting

Intermittent fasting has become quite popular, in large part, due to the many,different benefits it offers. Given its popularity, there are individual variations of this diet that have been conjured. All of these methods, if implemented correctly, can be equally useful. Which particular way of applying intermittent fasting works best depends on the goals that one has set for themselves.

16/8 Method

The 16/8 method is one of the most natural intermittent fasting protocols there is. It takes advantage of the fact that the normal human schedule leaves a person effectively fasting while asleep. This method is merely an extension of that fasting period. In this plan, most people skip breakfast and have their first meal after noon. The key to this method of fasting is to ensure that the eating window does not exceed eight hours. So in the aforementioned schedule, 8 o'clock would be the last time for eating anything. In this process, an individual is required to fast for sixteen hours a day. The eating window is restricted to eight hours. Two regular or three small meals can be squeezed into this period.

This method is quite simple to follow. It could be something as simple as skipping breakfast or not munching on anything after dinner. For instance, you can make sure that the last meal you have is at 8 in the evening. Then one needs to make sure not to eat anything until noon the following day. This provides a fasting window of about sixteen hours. As this configuration of intermittent fasting has been used and studied, it has been observed that it may be better for women to fast for a shorter duration of time, keeping their fasting period under 14-15 hours. For those who are used to having breakfast every day and feel hungry in the morning, this can be hard at first. Of course, for someone who is already used to skipping breakfast, it should be easy. While fasting, it is permissible to have water, coffee and other beverages without calories. For someone just getting started with intermittent fasting, the 16/8 method is the best fasting protocol to consider.

5:2 Method

For those who do not like the idea of fasting daily, the 5:2 protocol is another option. It is quite an easy way of fasting. The paradigm is fasting on two days of the week and eating like normal on the other five days. On the fasting days, men must ensure that their calorie intake does not exceed approximately six hundred calories. The calorie limit for women on fasting days is approximately five hundred calories. Obviously, these are estimates for an average-sized person of each respective gender. On fasting days, one can eat two meals consisting of 250-300 calories each, depending on gender. This nutritional schedule is suitable for all those who feel they cannot fast for the whole day and would like to eat a little something. The 5:2 protocol is a straightforward plan. It allows control over determining the days on which to fast and the days on which to eat normally. On the fasting days, there is the option to either stick to a strict fast or indulge in one meal around five hundred calories. If the idea of abstaining from eating is not attractive, then this plan is a great option.

Eat-Stop-Eat

This form of intermittent fasting requires the individual to fast for a full twenty-four hours, once or twice every week. That means not eating from dinner on one day until dinner the consecutive day. For instance, if lunch ended at 1 pm on Monday, then lunch on Tuesday should not come until 1 pm. That is the twenty-four hour fasting window. Which particular twenty-four hour period includes the fast is not important; the important part is that the fast lasts the full length of time in order to allow the body to run through its full beneficial process during fasting. The fast must be a complete fast, as well, without any solid food or caloric consumption. However, water, coffee and other beverages that don't have any calories in them can be safely consumed. Anyone following this method in order to lose weight needs to eat regularly during the feeding window.

The chief drawback to this method is the twenty-four-hour fasting window, which could prove difficult to follow. For that reason, the eat-stop-eat method may not be the best way to begin intermittent fasting. Fortunately, by beginning with the 16/8 method, there is only an additional eight hours needed to gradually progress to a twenty-four hour fasting window. The first stretch of the fast should not be any harder than usual; only towards the end of the twenty-four fast might this plan get especially challenging. That is where discipline and motivation come in.

One way to stay focused and committed during a fast is by keeping busy because it leaves little time to think about food or hunger. As a fasting day approaches, intentional efforts to plan activities can promote success during the fast. On the other hand, it is helpful to avoid planning a fast at the same times as social occasions, since fasting can put a damper on everyone's enjoyment of food and drink. Intermittent fasting protocols are quite convenient, and you shouldn't have to compromise on your social life for the sake of this diet.

Drinking plenty of water is another way to endure fasting. Not only will it provide by way of hydration for the body, but it will also take up space in the stomach and produce a full feeling for longer.

Warrior Diet

This kind of fasting involves the consumption of small quantities of raw fruit and vegetables during the day and then eating a single hearty meal at night. Mostly, it requires fasting throughout the day, and feasting at night. The feeding window recedes to only four hours. This variation of intermittent fasting was one of the first ones to be popular. While following this method of fasting, food choices should be quite similar to those eaten on the Paleo diet. That means consuming a high percentage of unprocessed foods. In fact, anything that humanity's cavemen ancestors would have eaten is acceptable. If something looks like it was produced in a factory, it should be avoided.

The Paleo diet is a high-fat and low-carb diet, just like the ketogenic diet. The protocols of a Paleo diet can be successfully combined with the protocols of an intermittent fast. For instance, if one follows the alternate day model of fasting, then the non-fasting days could follow a Paleo diet. No matter what, any food consumed must be Paleo-friendly. No form of processed foods, starchy foods, or carbs are permitted. Combining these two nutritional strategies can result in great benefits for both health and weight loss.

Multi-Day Fasting

While it may stretch the purview of focus on intermittent fasting—by definition not a prolonged fast—the health benefits of multi-day fasting are worth considering. With increased knowledge of one's body and its tendencies and successes in following a pattern of intermittent fasting, an occasion multi-day fast may offer helpful variety as well as physiological benefits.

The sweet spot for multi-day fasts, according to recent studies on maximizing the impact of autophagy, is twenty-four to forty-eight hours.[3] A 2010 study[4] in food-restricted mice found that autophagy increased significantly after the twenty-four hour mark. Gains were even more impressive another twenty-four hours later. There was also a possibility that the rate of autophagy grew even more after the forty-eight hour mark, but the study was not conclusive on that point.

For the purposes of practicing a multi-day fast, many people find the first three days to be the most difficult to endure, so if a sizable benefit is achievable at twenty-four hours with only a third of the misery, then there is a practical medium. That said, there is a long history of extended fasting within several various religious traditions. The forty-day fast of Jesus in the wilderness is a prime example. In more recent history, Mohandas Gandhi used food restriction as a means of nonviolent protest, enduring as long as twenty-one days without food[5].

Skipping Meals Spontaneously

For the spontaneous-minded, it is possible to enjoy the benefits of intermittent fasting without a structured plan. Essentially, spontaneous fasting involves skipping meals instinctively from time to time. Simply, if eating is not convenient or necessary, then it could be a good occasion to skip a meal. Some reasons for skipping a meal could include having little or no hunger, preoccupation with work or another activity, or not wanting to take the time and effort to prepare a healthy meal. The next meal can be a hearty one. One

---

[3] Levy, J. (2018, Apr. 9). Benefits of Authophagy, Plus How to Induce It. Retrieved from https://draxe.com/benefits-of-autophagy/
[4] Alirezaei, M., Kemball, C.C., Flynn, C.T., Wood, M.R., Whitton, J.L., & Kiosses, W.B. (2010). Short-term fasting induces profound neuronal autophagy. Retrieved from https://www.ncbi.nlm.nih.gov/pmc/articles/PMC3106288/
[5] Gandhi Begins Fast of 21 Days. (1943, Feb. 12). Retrieved from https://trove.nla.gov.au/newspaper/article/25940968

necessary caution about spontaneous fasting is that it does not become an occasion for eating unhealthily because of the lack of structure. Additionally, skipping meals is not the same as starvation. Starvation or anorexia is not what this method is about. The key to the strategy is avoiding meals out of habit or social conditioning. Instead, hunger becomes the main driver of food consumption. If hunger is minimal or non-existent, then there is an occasion for skipping a meal. The result is a reduction of unnecessary calorie consumption. The body knows what it needs – the challenge is learning to listen to it. Eating only when hungry will help.

Liquid Fast

Each of the methods above have to do with the structure of time with regards to the fast. With the exception of the Warrior Diet, none of them distinguishes the kinds of food that are eaten during periods of intake. A liquid fast differs from these other eating patterns in that it describes a method that is defined entirely by its nutritional content rather than by the duration or timing of feeding and fasting periods.

The liquid fast is fairly self-explanatory. In place of solid foods, liquids serve as the form of nutrition. These liquids can include broths (derived from meat and vegetables), juices, milk, yogurt, kefir, smoothies, avocado, certain types of tofu, and a range of other liquid, semi-liquid, or soft foods that can be transformed into think liquid form.[6] Typically, a liquid fast lasts for one to three days.

The identified benefits of a liquid fast or liquid diet are predictable. Weight loss occurs because of a reduction in calorie intake, oftentimes as much as a pound per day. When the liquids absorbed are high in vitamin and mineral content, there is a benefit to organ

---

[6] Staughton, J. (2019, Feb. 10). 5 Scientifically Proven Benefits of Liquid Diet. Retrieved from https://owl.purdue.edu/owl/research_and_citation/apa_style/apa_formatting_an d_style_guide/reference_list_electronic_sources.html

functioning. Perhaps the greatest benefit of a liquid diet is elimination of toxins. The body realizes energy savings because it does not have to work as hard digesting liquids as it would breaking down solids. The increase in energy is then available for the body's detoxifying of organs in order to cleanse the system. Toxins are flushed from the body by the abundance of liquid to carry it.

The downsides of a liquid diet are only serious with a prolonged avoidance of solid food. These complications include nutrient deficiency because of the limited array of foods enjoyed, constipation because of a lack of fiber, and a drop in muscle mass as the body begins to burn lean muscle in the absence of sufficient fuel.

Much like the ketogenic diet that will be featured in Chapter 7, a liquid diet is an option to complement a schedule of intermittent fasting. Because of its detoxifying effects, it could prove a helpful option to incorporate on a monthly or bi-weekly basis, substituting for either a fasting period or a feeding period. It might also be used as a transitional step when first initiating a full fast.

Chapter Three:

How to Go About Intermittent Fasting

Selecting a method

It is essential that each individual chooses a method that suits his or her needs and requirements. Doing this increases the chances of success while following this diet. Selecting an ideal way not only increases the likelihood of fasting effectively, but it also reduces the possibility of giving up. If the selected method fits seamlessly into one's lifestyle, then adherence to the plan is more likely. If the protocol doesn't fit in, then it will only cause additional stress, and stress reduces the chances of following the diet.

When it comes to selecting a method of intermittent fasting, there are a couple of different things to consider. Given the fact that there are various options available, how does one pick the diet that best suits their needs? The remainder of this chapter presents several questions to consider when deciding upon the best method of intermittent fasting.

What constitutes a regular diet?

If one's regular diet is full of processed foods, carbs and sugars, then fasting might not be as easy. A diet that is rich in sugar is somewhat addictive and letting go of this addiction may take some time. Beginning an intermittent fasting protocol like the 16/8 method or even the twenty-four-hour fasting method will likely surface symptoms of sugar withdrawal. When this happens, the chances of quitting the regimen increase tremendously. The solution is to opt for a diet and intake plan that isn't too extreme – at least to start.

There is wisdom in slowly getting one's body accustomed to the new regimen. With a baseline established, it becomes much easier to make gradual, specific changes that will make the transition into a new eating plan simpler. For instance, if one's regular menu is heavy on carbohydrates, then a strategy of slowly eliminating some of the more processed carbs is advisable. Perhaps cutting out one type of carb from the diet every two days would be a sufficient way to proceed. Soon the diet will consist of only healthy foods, with no binging on unhealthy items.

If one's eating schedule consists of frequent consumption, then a slow reduction in the number of snacks in between meals will help establish a course of intermittent fasting. With snacking eliminated, the next step is to slowly increase the duration of time between meals. Doing all this will slowly condition the body for fasting.

An immediate radical approach does not benefit the body, so starting slowly is an important strategy for success. It is possible to take full advantage of intermittent fasting without causing harmful hormonal disturbances in the body. And by following the protocols of intermittent fasting correctly, losing extra pounds is not only possible, but likely.

What thoughts or beliefs does fasting inspire?

For any discipline to be successful, the subject must be invested in that discipline – both physically and psychologically. Thinking that fasting is not possible, or having a belief that fasting is scary significantly lessens the chances of success. Trying a new nutritional plan requires open-mindedness about the foods involved and the schedule for eating. It also requires trust in the plan.

What does an average day look like?

Before selecting the ideal method of fasting, one must look closely at his or her daily schedule. For instance, someone used to waking up early in the morning who likes to exercise is already well-suited to the 16/8 method. Someone who does not have the time to eat three meals a day and prefers a couple of light snacks during the day and a heavy dinner at night should opt for the Warrior Diet. The bottom line is that the method of fasting chosen must be easy to follow, and it should easily fit into one's daily schedule without causing any additional stress.

Which drinks are OK during a fast?

Consuming drinks is fine while fasting, as long as these drinks are calorie-free. Regardless of the preferred method of fasting, it will always be helpful to have certain fasting-friendly beverages handy. Such aids will not only reinforce the diet thorough hydration, but they will also reduce hunger pangs. The big question, then, is what specifically can one drink during fasting without ruining the effects of the fast? The items specified in this section will help increase the efficiency of the fast and will also help with gut health.

Herbal Teas
Tea can be enjoyed without restriction or limitation, so long as there are no sweeteners or milk added to it. The best options available are herbal teas. Herbal teas have plenty of benefits, and they also help keep hunger pangs at bay. Different herbal teas have different effects on the body. For instance, a cup of chamomile tea can produce a calming effect, and a cup of peppermint tea can be refreshing and energizing.

Coffee
A person fasting can drink unsweetened coffee without any milk or cream added to it. Caffeine not only provides an instant burst of energy, but it also helps regulate hunger pangs. Like anything,

coffee should be consumed in moderation. Too much caffeine is not a good thing, and unregulated coffee intake could result in negative health consequences.

Baking Soda

Baking soda is commonly used in cooking, but it has several health benefits to offer. It helps with several digestive issues like constipation and bloating. It helps kill any harmful bacteria as well as parasites present in the gut. It helps reduce fatigue and tiredness of muscles. It stabilizes the pH level of the stomach and neutralizes acidity. Take a glass of water and add a teaspoon of baking soda to ensure that electrolyte levels in the body are balanced.

Artificial Sweeteners

Beverages that contain any form of artificial sweeteners should be avoided during a fasting regimen. Consumption of preprocessed and prepackaged drinks should be considered as a break in a fast. The common types of artificial sweeteners are maltodextrin, dextrose, and sucralose. All these sweeteners contain some carbs, and consuming any of them during the fasting period will disrupt the impact of fasting upon the body. Just one weak moment can negate all of the discipline and effort that has gone into a fast. Natural sweeteners like stevia are acceptable to sweeten any beverages. However, it is important to observe any impacts of natural sweeteners on the body before drinking too much of any natural sweetener.

Glauber's Salts

If one's primary reason for fasting is to promote cellular health and improve overall health, then consuming Glauber's salts during the fasting window is a good idea. It is usually known as sodium sulfate decahydrate. Glauber's salts are used as a mild laxative, meaning they help with bowel movements. However, please note that consuming more than twenty grams of Glauber's salts in a day can induce diarrhea, so just be cautious of how much you are consuming.

Apple Cider Vinegar
Apple cider vinegar helps keep hunger pangs at bay, cleanses the gut, and even provides an instant energy boost. The acidic elements present in it help regulate the body's pH levels. Apple cider vinegar can be added to water or taken by itself a tablespoon at a time. It is entirely up to preference.

Water
Drinking plenty of water makes skin clearer and flushes out many toxins from the body. Drinking at least eight glasses of water daily on average should be a habit. Providing some variation with flavorings or electrolytes to your water can spruce it up. Slices of lemon, different berries, a handful of mint leaves, or slices of cucumber can be added to water to further body detoxification while adding flavor. Following these simple tips can boost water intake.

Drinking water needs to be convenient, too. If water is not available, it cannot be consumed. Carrying a water bottle or a sipper at all times guarantees a constant supply. If a water bottle is handy, it is more likely that you will drink water without a reminder. Forming habits, like drinking a glass of water before and after each meal, can make it easier to reach the quota for each day. Some people will also be motivated by setting a daily water consumption goal and tracking progress toward the goal. Keeping track of intake produces natural motivation to drink more. It is difficult to overstate the value of staying well hydrated, since water is an essential ingredient in most body processes. It is a basic strategy for health and wellness.

Chapter Four:

Intermittent Fasting and Weight Loss

Intermittent fasting can lead to dramatic weight loss, which is one of its most appealing and tangible benefits — as long as it is done in a healthy way. The reasons for weight loss range from hormonal changes, improved metabolic rate, reduced consumption, and behavioral changes.

Fasting for short periods helps optimize the hormones that regulate weight gain or loss. The body stores away energy or calories in the form of body fat. When no new fuel comes into the body, then the body changes several things within itself to make this stored energy available to it. Basically, the major internal changes the body makes relate to activities performed by the central nervous system and the levels of various essential hormones. When nutrients enter the body's digestive system, insulin levels increase. In the absence of such nutrients, insulin levels decrease. With a low level of insulin, the body will begin burning away accumulated fat. The result is weight loss through reduction of fat tissue and a body that becomes more lean.

Another factor in promoting leanness is Human Growth Hormone, or HGH. During a fast, HGH increases, and this helps in gaining muscle and reducing fat. Fat cells are broken down into norepinephrine, and this helps in the burning of fatty acids for generating energy. Even without any increase in muscle mass, the burning of fat would still result in a higher ratio of muscle to fat, or a more lean body type. However, there are even more benefits to enjoy because of the impact of HGH.

In short, intermittent fasting can actually increase muscle mass. That might seem counter-intuitive, since the stereotype of bodybuilders and high-performance athletes is that they consume ten thousand calories a day, eating frequently to fuel the constant repair and building up of muscle tissue. Should not the opposite be true, as well, that if one restricts intake of nutrients, then muscle mass will diminish? Studies have repeatedly demonstrated that intermittent fasting can help you shed weight without any reduction in muscle mass. On a diet based solely on caloric restrictions, the body starts breaking down muscle to fuel itself. In heavy caloric restriction diets, about twenty-five percent of the weight shed comes from muscle mass. Yet in intermittent fasting diets, only ten percent of weight loss was attributed to loss of muscle mass. (This is one reason why most intermittent fasting guidelines recommend taking up strength training, to minimize muscle loss and instead take advantage of the presence of HGH to build muscle through exercise). Furthermore, one study required the participants to consume the same amount of calories, except they had to do this in just one huge meal given to them in the evening. They not only lost body fat but also increased their muscle build up, along with a host of other beneficial changes to their health. When compared to any standard diet, intermittent fasting will preserve muscle mass while burning away unnecessary body fat.

Transforming a flabby, soft body into a lean, tight body leads to additional gains that help with continuous fat burning and maintaining weight loss. Sinewy lean muscle that comes from strength training and HGH production is more metabolically active than fat tissue. That lean body type will have a higher basal metabolic rate (BMR), the aspect of the body's metabolism that is responsible for as much as eighty percent of calorie burning.[7] A further metabolic benefit of intermittent fasting versus simple calorie reduction diets is that BMR has been shown to stay constant during intermittent fasting, while traditional restriction diets result in lowered BMR.[8] When people lose weight on calorie-restriction diets, they end up losing significant amounts of muscle mass, leading to a lower metabolic rate, and weight that was lost begins to accumulate once more. The result is the familiar "boomerang effect" of rapidly losing and then regaining weight, a phenomenon of so many fad and crash diets. By contrast, the comparably higher metabolic rate associated with intermittent fasting means that weight lost stays off. The higher BMR enables faster burning of calories and fat cells during fasting.

While the impact is probably minimal, intermittent fasting may assist weight loss by reducing calorie intake. Intermittent fasting is indeed a convenient way of restricting calories consumed without requiring any conscious effort of trying to eat less. The different protocols for fasting ensure that calorie consumption is not higher than what is required by the body. Eating twice a day instead of three times should result in less caloric consumption, on average. Alternate day fasting has been shown to reduce 1.7 pounds every week. There is a clear benefit, then, to intermittent fasting. But attributing those benefits to reduced calorie consumption misses the mark. Ultimately, fasting has very little to do with calories. The

---

[7] Julia Belluz reports that rates of calorie burning for BMR range from sixty-five to eighty percent for adults. (2018). What I learned about weight loss from spending a day inside a metabolic chamber. Retrieved from https://www.vox.com/2018/9/4/17486110/metabolism-diet-fast-weight-loss

[8] "In other words, what the study shows is if you simply cut your calories, your metabolic rate is going to go down and that's [00:03:00] bad because you're not burning as much calories. If you do the fasting, on the other hand, there's no statistically significant drop in your basal metabolic rate, which is good because now, one, you've switched over to burning fat, but you're burning it at the same rate you were before." Fong, J. [Transcript of podcast.] Retrieved from https://idmprogram.com/wp-content/uploads/Episode-14-Science-Transcript.pdf.

most important element of fasting that makes it effective is time spent not eating. That's when the hormonal changes occur that promote permanent weight loss.

On the other hand, a non-physiological benefit that can have varying degrees of impact upon weight loss is the behavioral change associated with intermittent fasting. The necessary attention toward eating patterns, types of nutrition, hydration, and exercise – mindfulness about health — can promote healthier habits. Someone who is fasting will be more likely to consume high-quality food, including whole foods whenever possible. The discipline of abiding by planned feeding and fasting times also contributes to weight loss. Binging on junk food during a fast period is a sure way to reduce or eliminate gains. Compensating afterward for calories unconsumed during a fast period will also limit the effectiveness of the fasting plan. Restraint and discipline will help achieve the maximum benefit of intermittent fasting. Being consistent is essential. Especially in the early going, it is important to trust the process and persist despite the discomfort of hunger pangs. After three weeks of following intermittent fasting, changes in bodily appearance and weight should be apparent. Quitting before that point would prevent someone from seeing those emerging results. Even after that point, it is important to remain patient and disciplined. The crucial processes are taking place internally. It takes time to get used to this kind of life change – physically as well as psychologically. Consistency with meal schedules is vital, and over a period of time, this can become easy.

At the end of the day, losing weight is only one of the many benefits of intermittent fasting. Intermittent fasting is a highly effective means of losing weight, but its benefits go well beyond mere weight loss.

Chapter Five:

Fasting and Human Growth Hormone

The last chapter explained in brief that fasting increases Human Growth Hormone (HGH), which has a key role in muscle building and fat burning. There are additional benefits from natural HGH production that enhance the long-term value of intermittent fasting, including anti-aging properties. Before turning to those concerns, a basic understanding of HGH's interactions will be helpful.

HGH is produced by the body's master gland, the pituitary gland. This gland plays a vital role in the development and growth of children and adolescents. HGH levels spike up during puberty and start decreasing after that. But its importance does not end there. It plays an active role in the health of adults as well. A deficiency in HGH in an adult may lead to an increase in the level of body fat, reduce lean body mass, and hurt bone mass. Once HGH has been released by the pituitary gland, it is present in the bloodstream for only a couple of minutes. It is then transported to the liver, and then converted into a variety of growth factors. The most important of all is Insulin-Like Growth Factor 1, also known as IGF1. It is involved in the growth, development, and maintenance of several various organs and body systems.

The growth hormone is a counter-regulatory hormone, and it is secreted during sleep. HGH coupled with cortisol and adrenaline helps in increasing the levels of glucose in the blood by breaking down the glycogen present in it. This helps in countering the effect of insulin. These hormones are usually secreted just before waking up, around 4 am or so. The burst of HGH helps the body to prepare itself for a long day of work. It pushes out some glucose from the storage compartment in the body and into the bloodstream – thereby making it available for providing energy.

When people say that it is necessary to have a hearty breakfast to keep them going throughout the day, they cannot be farther away from the truth. The human body has already given itself a good boost of necessary energy, and it is charged up to get through the day ahead. There is no need to binge on carbs or any sugary cereals to provide the body with the energy it needs. This is also a reason for the lack of hunger in the morning. Even though the body has not consumed anything for ten hours or so, there is usually little desire to eat in the morning. The body has already given itself the energy boost it needs. Despite the flawed conventional wisdom that breakfast is the most important meal of the day[9], eating a hearty breakfast only serves to dump unnecessary calories—normally empty calories from convenient processed foods—into the bloodstream.

HGH for Anti-Aging

The secretion of HGH decreases with age, and if its level is abnormally low, then it will likely lead to a reduction in muscle and bone mass. In 1990, a study was conducted regarding the effect of giving HGH to people who were old and had very low levels of HGH. The study's participants were divided into two groups. The first group was given HGH and the second group got none. The study was conducted over the course of six months. There was no change

---

[9] It's been fairly well documented that the campaign in support of breakfast was not steeped in objectivity, as General Mills and Kraft sponsored a third of the studies. One such example is Stossel, J. (2019). Forget the hype; breakfast isn't important. Retrieved from
https://www.palmbeachdailynews.com/article/20190411/OPINION/190419494.

in the overall weight of either of these groups. However, there was a significant difference in lean body mass. The HGH group had gained, on average, 3.7 kilograms in the form of lean mass. That's about eight pounds of lean mass. The fat mass also decreased by about five pounds. The health of the subjects' skin improved, as well. The recipients of HGH not only lost unnecessary fat but gained lean muscle. In an article that was published in 2002 in JAMA, similar results were obtained from the experiment when conducted on women.

This does sound pretty good...so, why isn't everyone using this? Well, for starters, these studies show the results of HGH when used on a person with a low level of HGH. It wasn't tested for people with a reasonable degree of HGH, because there would be an increase in the level of blood sugars. This would make sense because HGH is a counter-regulatory hormone. Pre-diabetes would increase because of this. This, in turn, would lead to fluid retention and an increase in the levels of blood pressure. In the long run, this would lead to several other health problems as well. So, that isn't good news. Artificial injections of HGH are not a viable option. However, what if there was a natural method for increasing this hormone?

Fasting for Increasing HGH

In 1982[10], a study was published that described a single participant who had decided to undergo a forty-day fast for religious reasons. During the forty days, the subject's glucose level dropped from 96 to 56. This, in turn, led to a drastic drop in their level of insulin (from 13.5 to 2.91)[11]. The primary interest in this study came about when an increase in HGH levels was discovered. The HGH level started at 0.73 and increased to 9.86. That's a significant increase in the level of

---

[10] Kerndt, P.R., Naughton, J.L., Driscoll, C.E., & Loxterkamp, D.A. (1982 Nov.). Fasting: the history, pathophysiology and complications. Retrieved from https://www.ncbi.nlm.nih.gov/pubmed/6758355
[11] Such data shows the great promise fasting offers for those suffering with Type 2 diabetes.

growth hormone without the use of any pharmaceuticals. Additionally, there seemed to be no side effects to this spike. The levels of glucose and blood pressure appeared to be well balanced. There have been other studies that have shown a similar, natural increase in the levels of HGH through fasting. In 1988, KY Ho, et al.[12] studied fasting and HGH. They concluded that consumption of food helps in suppressing the level of HGH. This is naturally expected. Just like cortisol, HGH increases the level of glucose, and this tends to get crushed during the feeding period. Fasting helps in stimulating the secretion of HGH. During the fasting period, there is a spike in the flow of HGH in the morning. However, it is regularly secreted even throughout the day.

HGH and Musculoskeletal Mass

One major misconception that a lot of people have about fasting is that it leads to a reduction in lean mass. They draw this conclusion, which seems logical, from the assumption that a lack of fuel and nutrients will rob the body of the raw material it needs to build and sustain its mass. However, this cannot be farther away from the truth.

HGH is the key hormone that preserves bone mass and muscle mass. Fasting, rather than reducing HGH levels, instead boosts this builder of the human musculoskeletal organs. Fasting is better at preserving lean mass when compared to other diets that prescribe intense caloric reduction. There seems to be an evolutionary basis to this phenomenon in the human body. During summers in the Paleolithic era, the early man would eat lots of food, and those nutrients would be stored as fat within the cells of his body, to be

---

[12] Ho, K.Y., Veldhuis, J.D., Johnson, M.L., Furlanetto, R., Evans, W.S., Alberti, K.G., & Thorner, M.O. (1988). Fasting enhances growth hormone secretion and amplifies the complex rhythms of growth hormone secretion in man. Retrieved from https://www.ncbi.nlm.nih.gov/pubmed/3127426

burned for energy during the lean and unproductive winter. So, what exactly would his constitution do? Would it start burning muscle instead of burning all that stored fat? All the fat stored in your body is the reserve for much-needed energy. This is similar to you stocking up on firewood for your wood-burning stove. You have packed your storage unit with all the firewood it needs and then some. There's so much stocked up, that it is spilling out and you don't have room for all the wood that's boarded up. So, in times of need, would you use all this wood or chop up your table and throw it on the stove? That sounds rather silly, doesn't it? The same goes for your body as well. It starts by burning out all the fat that is stored in its reserves. Only after all this fat has been exhausted will your body burn muscle. However, with intermittent fasting, it certainly shouldn't come to this. The spike in the secretion of HGH helps in maintaining lean mass even while fasting.

Chapter Six:

Common FAQs

Since adopting a regimen of intermittent fasting may represent a drastic life change for many people, there is value in addressing some of the most frequently asked questions related to it.

How long does it take to get used to fasting?

It normally takes the body a week or two to get used to intermittent fasting. One way to help ease the transition is to make sure that exercise is not too stressful during the first two weeks. Afterwards, based on how things feel, continuing with life as normal should be fine.

Doesn't constant snacking help manage hunger?

It is a popular myth that eating frequently helps in keeping hunger and cravings at bay. However, this isn't necessarily true. If someone keeps increasing the amount of food they consume, then their need for the same will increase too. A couple of studies show that increasing the frequency of meals will lead to a reduction in hunger, some other studies recorded no change, and some suggest that there can be an increase in the hunger levels of an individual. One study showed that consuming three meals that are rich in protein are better at reducing hunger than consuming six small meals that are rich in protein. In other words, there is no proof at all that constant snacking keeps hunger at bay.

Isn't it necessary to eat every couple of hours to maintain stable blood sugar levels?

No, it is not necessary to keep eating regularly. Unless someone suffers from hypoglycemia, they do not have to worry about feeling weak or dizzy without eating every couple of hours. Skipping breakfast certainly does not cause any harm. A healthy body can maintain itself without food for prolonged periods of time. Intermittent fasting does not prescribe starvation. It merely asks the individual to employ fasting for a certain period of time before food consumption.

Will fasting lead to an increase in fat storage?

With the introduction of more nutrients every couple of hours, it is very difficult for the body to burn any fat. The body's preference is to burn glucose, the sugar that is readily available from recently consumed food, especially carbohydrates. When those nutrients are available, the body will not burn anything else. With a steady influx of fuel, the body will not get a chance to burn the fat stored within cells. Even more, whatever newly introduced nutrients are not immediately burned are themselves converted to fat. As a consequence, fat loss and related weight loss never occurs. So regular and steady intake of food actually leads to an increase in fat storage.

Fasting, by contrast, helps to decrease insulin levels, and it promotes lipolysis. Lipolysis is the process by which the body starts to burn the fat that it has stored. When the body enters a fasted state, it starts to burn fat. When the next meal introduces new nutrients into the body, the body stops burning fat and concentrates only on breaking down the food consumed at the moment. Because of the body's tendency to switch into lipolysis, there is no need to worry about the body's metabolism slowing down.

Will the body enter into starvation mode?

According to different claims, not consuming food will make one's body feel that it is starving. This, in turn, is said to shut down its metabolic functions and hinder it from burning fat. Long-term starvation can indeed reduce the burning of calories in the body. This is referred to as starvation mode or thermogenesis. Depending upon the intake of calories, the body will decide how many calories it can afford to burn. Thermogenesis is inevitable when it comes to weight loss. However, no valid evidence suggests that thermogenesis is a common state for the body during intermittent fasting. Fasting for short periods will help to increase the metabolic rate of the body. During a short-term fast, there is a spike in the levels of norepinephrine or noradrenaline. This, in turn, helps in breaking down fat and promoting a faster metabolism.

What foods are best to eat while fasting?

There are not any dietary restrictions per se on an intermittent fast.

The chief principle is to be mindful of eating times. What one eats is of less concern. However, the benefits of fasting do not offer license to fast for sixteen hours and then fill up with all sorts of processed junk food. That kind of undisciplined behavior will only defeat the purpose of fasting. There are no dietary restrictions, and there is no need to count calories, but that does not mean that one should eat unhealthily. The goal should be to eat well-balanced meals that are full of a wide range of necessary nutrients and dietary fiber. Healthy meals must be rich in protein, dietary fats, and fiber.

Can intermittent fasting be combined with any other diet?

Intermittent fasting is one of the most versatile dieting protocols, and combining intermittent fasting with other dieting protocols can speed up the process of weight loss. Intermittent fasting can easily be coupled with other diets like the ketogenic diet and the paleo diet.

A ketogenic diet is a low-carb, high-fat diet in which the body produces ketones for providing energy, hence its name. The body produces ketones when there is a reduction in the consumption of carbs. When carb consumption is reduced, the body reaches into its reserves of fat for generating energy. Intermittent fasting protocols can be easily combined with the ketogenic diet. One important consideration is that during the eating window, the food that is consumed should have a high fat content and low or no carbs.

Another diet that intermittent fasting can be efficiently combined with is the Paleo diet. The Paleo diet is a low-carb high-fat diet like the ketogenic diet. However, the Paleo diet permits only such foods as would have been available in the Paleolithic era. This diet prohibits the consumption of all grains, processed foods, sugars, and anything that human beings produce by making use of machines. Whether from following one of these diets or by simply eating a menu rich in whole foods, intermittent fasting's weight loss and health benefits can become more effective when combined with purposeful selection of foods.

What are the side effects of this eating plan?

There are not any severe or worrying side effects of intermittent fasting. Most commonly, people feel light-headed and might experience mild headaches. However, this is a sign that the body is getting used to intermittent fasting. It is not something to worry about.

To ensure optimal health, there are several things that can be done:

- Stay thoroughly hydrated.

- Be attentive to your body's warning signs.

- Breaking the fast is not the worst thing, as long as it is not a regular occurrence. There are some days and times when the body's nutritional needs vary, and it is fine to respond to the signs of those needs.

Is fasting harmful to one's health?

One of the apparent drawbacks about intermittent fasting is that there is limited scientific and statistical data about it, especially longitudinal studies to show the long-term effects. There is, then, a possibility that some detriment lies undetected. On the other hand, fasting generally, and intermittent fasting specifically, has a long track record of use throughout history. A lack of scientific and statistical data may not be necessary to establish the validity of a practice that has been tried and tested for generations.

Frame of reference is important to this question, as well. The modern era of human society in the developed nations of the world is laden with excess and abundance, in many cases. In such contexts, a lifestyle like intermittent fasting may seem extreme or needlessly difficult. Yet in developing nations, it is a necessity and not a luxury of choice, much as it has been for the majority of humanity throughout history.

Finally, to evaluate intermittent fasting based on currently observable phenomena, it appears to have extreme benefits. However, it is important to note that fasting is a stressor to the body; it releases the stress hormone cortisol into the body. Similar to something like weight training, intermittent fasting is beneficial to a point, but could be detrimental if overdone. Misuse or abuse does not make something inherently bad. Intermittent fasting and working out are both great, powerful, and beneficial things — when implemented properly.

Will intermittent fasting cause thyroid problems or make them worse?

Because the thyroid gland plays such an important role in regulating metabolism and organ function, it is an important question whether fasting disrupts its functioning or effectiveness. This is especially true because of fasting's obvious impact upon metabolism.

Multi-day fasting has a clear impact on the hormone secretions of the thyroid, particularly thyroid hormone T3.[13] Other hormones, including thyroid hormone T4 and the thyroid stimulating hormone do not change. In the studies that bear out those conclusions, participants were subjected to conditions more closely related to starvation than intermittent fasting, though. Solomon therefore concludes that the impact upon T3 (and the other thyroid hormones studied) during intermittent fasting is minimal.[14]

The nutrient iodine is crucial to production of thyroid hormone. For adults, the end result can be hypothyroidism. The consequences are much more dire for children and fetuses. So the greatest risk for the thyroid for someone following a pattern of intermittent fasting is simple iodine deficiency. Yet for someone practicing intermittent fasting with a reasonably varied palate, iodine deficiency is highly unlikely. There is no evidence, then, that intermittent fasting could in and of itself cause thyroid dysfunction.

But is intermittent fasting safe for someone who already has problems with thyroid function? Even for perfectly healthy people, consulting with a physician is a wise precaution before beginning

---

[13] Solomon, S. (2015, Aug. 2). Fasting and Thyroid. Retrieved from https://www.drsarasolomon.com/fasting-and-thyroid/
Tabor, V.H. (2018, Oct. 19). Intermittent fasting, your thyroid, and your immune system. Retrieved from https://medium.com/boosted/intermittent-fasting-your-thyroid-and-your-immune-system-ec8f5f02d997
[14] Solomon.

any dramatic treatment or health-related life change. With that caveat, there is evidence that intermittent fasting can actually provide relief and improve the functioning of an unhealthy thyroid.

Based on the premise that fasting makes the human body more responsive to its hormones, Dr. Daniel Pompa advocates for using fasting as a means of improving the thyroid's functionality.[15] He cites fasting's unparalleled speed in reducing cellular inflammation as an important vehicle to stimulate healing and restore proper function to the thyroid. He lays out a diet and fasting regimen that ensures an adequate store of the nutrients needed to produce thyroid hormones while also taking advantage of the best elements of fasting. His basic week consists of three days of intermittent fasting, two days of famine (only water), and two days of feasting. The key marker that he tracks to ensure the body is headed in the right direction is glucose, which should remain low enough for autophagy to occur. He also wants to focus on ketones increasing. That balance ensures enough insulin in the system to aid in the conversion of thyroid hormone T4 to T3 while providing the best environment for a degraded thyroid to heal itself.

Doesn't eating frequently help to boost metabolism?

People tend to believe that consuming small meals frequently will help in improving the body's metabolic rate. It is true that the body does make use of some energy for digestion and assimilation of the nutrients present in food. This is referred to as the thermic effect of food or TEF. It accounts for about twenty to thirty percent of the calories for burning protein, around ten percent for carbs and about three percent for fat. The TEF can account for ten percent of the total caloric value of the food consumed. The number of calories

---

[15] He details a "multi-therapeutic approach (including fasting) in Pompa, D. (2018, Sept. 11). Fasting and Thyroid Conditions: Is it Possible? Retrieved from https://drpompa.com/fasting-diet/fasting-thyroid-conditions/

you consume matter and not the number of meals you consume. Consuming six meals comprising of five hundred calories each would have the same effect as consuming three meals of one thousand calories each. The thermic effect would be about ten percent on average. This results in the burning of three hundred calories in either of the cases.

Does intermittent fasting lead to overeating?

Some claims have been made that intermittent fasting will not be of any help toward shedding weight because it causes the individual to overeat during the feeding window. This isn't entirely incorrect. It is partially correct that people tend to feel extremely hungry after they break their fast. However, these claims imply that people would feel the need to compensate for all the calories that they didn't consume throughout the day. However, this picture of compensation is not a complete one. A study shows that people who have fasted for one whole day end up consuming five hundred extra calories the following day. But if the standard caloric intake for a day is two thousand calories, then there is a net reduction of fifteen hundred calories. That is still a win. As one can see, intermittent fasting clearly helps in reducing one's overall intake of food. More importantly, it enhances the body's efficiency and boosts metabolism. It does not increase weight, rather it helps to decrease it. Once someone gets used to eating at particular time intervals, they learn to control their hunger, and fasting will help them lose weight.

Doesn't the brain need a constant supply of glucose?

Many people do believe that not eating carbs frequently will hinder the functioning of our brains. This is based on the popular misconception that the brain can function only by making use of glucose. However, one important fact is often left out of this equation. The body can efficiently manufacture glucose through a process referred to as gluconeogenesis[16]. The body stores glycogen in the liver and this can always be accessed for supplying the brain with the energy that it needs. The body produces ketones during a low-carb diet or extended periods of fasting. The body then switches the energy requirement of the brain from glucose to ketones. So, during a long fast, you need not worry about the brain not being able to support itself on glucose. The brain can make use of ketones through a process referred to as ketosis. In ketosis, glucose is produced from burning fats and proteins. Anyone who suffers from hypoglycemia must make sure to meet the required intake of carbs.

What are some other advantages of intermittent fasting?

Some people think that fasting may be harmful to their overall wellbeing. This is nothing but a myth. Intermittent fasting has many health benefits. For instance, it helps in changing the expression of specific genes that help in improving longevity and providing better protection against diseases. It also provides a boost to your metabolism and reduces oxidative stress in your body. Like mentioned earlier, it also helps in tackling inflammation and reducing the different risk factors for various heart diseases and conditions. Intermittent fasting could be amazing for your brain's wellbeing. It helps to increase the production of BDNF. BDNF stands for brain-derived neurotrophic factor. This helps in protecting you from the onset or progression of certain mental illnesses. People might think that fasting is harmful. However, the multiple advantages it offers make it quite appealing.

Beyond the health benefits, there is a great deal of convenience and flexibility to be gained from not having to eat as frequently. For instance, on the standard 16/8 diet, there is no worry about having to

[16] Berg, J., Tymoczko, J., & Stryer, L. (2019). Glucose Can Be Synthesized from Noncarbohydrate Precursors. Retrieved from https://www.ncbi.nlm.nih.gov/books/NBK22591/

prepare breakfast in the morning. That frees up at least an additional fifteen minutes for a longer shower, a quick strength-building workout, or some extra sleep (over the course of a week, fifteen minutes a day results in more than an hour and a half of additional sleep). In the case of fasting days, the benefits are even greater, either in the area of time saved both preparing and eating meals or in cost savings from not paying to eat out. Fasting provides flexibility and convenience.

The one last but simple benefit is that hunger, by contrast, results in the greater delight and enjoyment of food ("absence makes the heart grow fonder," as the expression goes). When consuming three, four, five, or six meals and snacks a day, the stomach and taste buds never clear the deck and develop true desire for wholesome nutrition. Learning and experiencing this has been one of the great joys of intermittent fasting that I've been able to experience myself!

Chapter Seven:

Fasting and The Ketogenic Diet

About the Ketogenic Diet

All the carbohydrates that the body ingests are broken down into simple sugars. This sugar is absorbed into the bloodstream and causes a spike in the levels of glucose. The body starts producing insulin to counteract the rise in glucose levels. Insulin is a fat storing hormone and is secreted by the pancreas. When insulin is produced in large amounts, it stops the body from burning fat, and all the fat is stored in the body cells. After a while, the body assumes that there is a shortage of essential nutrients and it causes hunger pangs and cravings for all sorts of carbohydrate and sugar-rich foods. Those signals make the body want to eat again, and this vicious cycle keeps going on and on. Restricting carbohydrate consumption causes blood sugar levels to stabilize, and there is less need for insulin. Furthermore, this leads to the burning of fats for providing energy, leading to fat loss.

The body favors glucose instead of fats, and it is stored in the liver. However, only a finite amount of glucose can be stored there. The rest is stored in the form of fat, and the storage space for fats is not restricted. This leads to the accumulation of fatty cells. When carbohydrate consumption is restricted, the production of glucose reduces as well, and the body automatically shifts to the next available source of energy – fat. Low-carb and high-fat diets like the keto diet make it easy for the body to reach into its fat reserves to provide energy. Since these fat reserves are not blocked by excess insulin, the body starts feeling fuller as well. Even when someone eats to their heart's content on a keto diet, calorie intake is bound to reduce. So there is no need to worry about calorie counting.

Carbohydrates are the main culprit. Thus, instead of trying to avoid fats, paying attention to the carbohydrates consumed is more important. Bread, pasta, rice, potatoes, and all other starchy foods should be avoided or limited.

Food List

Eat freely
Protein:

Grass-fed meats like beef, lamb, goat, and venison. Fish that is caught in the wild. Pastured pork, poultry, and eggs. Offal is edible too, but only if it is grass-fed.

Healthy fats:

All saturated fats like lard, tallow, chicken, duck, goose, ghee, butter, coconut oil, avocado oil, macadamia oil, olive oil, and any other monounsaturated fats. Polyunsaturated fats (of animal origin) like fatty fish and other seafood rich in Omega-3 are beneficial.

Non-starchy vegetables:

All sorts of green leafy vegetables like spinach, lettuce, chives, radicchio, bok choy, and the like. Cruciferous vegetables like kale, kohlrabi, and radish. Other vegetables like asparagus, cucumbers, zucchini, spaghetti squash, bamboo shoots, and celery.

Beverages and condiments:

Black coffee, black tea, green tea, any other herbal teas and the most obvious one – water. Bone broth is nourishing and filling.

Condiments like mayonnaise, pesto, mustard, pickles and fermented foods like kimchi, and sauerkraut (provided it is made at home). Use of spices and herbs for flavoring food can be used liberally.

Eat occasionally
Vegetables and fruits:

Specific cruciferous vegetables like white and red cabbage, cauliflower, broccoli, fennel, turnips, swede, and Brussels sprouts. Nightshades like eggplants, tomatoes, and different peppers. Few root vegetables like spring onions, parsley root, garlic, mushrooms, pumpkin, and leeks. Other vegetables like nori, okra, sugar snap peas, bean sprouts, wax beans, water chestnuts, and artichokes. Berries such as cranberries, blackberries, blueberries, raspberries, strawberries, and so on.

Dairy products:

Full-fat cream, yogurt, sour cream, cottage cheese (stay away from "low-fat" and "diet" products).

Nuts and seeds:

Macadamia nuts, pecans, almonds, walnuts, Brazil nuts, sunflower seeds, pine nuts, flaxseeds, pumpkin seeds, sesame seeds, and hemp seeds.

Fermented soy products:

Soy products without GMO like tempeh, soy sauce, and any other soy-based products. Edamame and unprocessed black soybeans.

Foods to avoid
The keto diet does not permit any grains, and this includes whole grains like wheat, rye, corn, barley, millets, sorghum, rice, buckwheat, etc. Therefore all foods from grain, like pasta, pizza,

bread, etc., are strictly prohibited. Pork and fish that have been farmed in factories containing high levels of Omega-6 fatty acids and mercury should be avoided. All sugary treats must be avoided, like sodas, ice creams, sugary syrups, and cakes.

Processed foods that contain carrageenan and MSG. No dried fruits and wheat gluten. Stay away from artificial sweeteners like Splenda, Equal, and all other sweeteners containing saccharin, sucralose, and aspartame. Read the labels carefully before picking up a sweetener. Refined fats, oils, and trans fats like margarine are restricted. Do not use sunflower oil, cottonseed oil, canola oil, corn oil, grapeseed oil, and soybean oil.

All products labeled as "low fat," "low carb," "zero-carb," and "diet" contain artificial additives and are not healthy.

Milk is allowed as long as it is full-fat. However, it easy to overlook the presence of carbohydrates because they are present in more than just starchy foods.

Tropical fruits like pineapple, mangoes, papayas, and bananas are prohibited. Fruits rich in carbs like tangerines and grapes must also be avoided. Avoid consuming any fruit juices, even the ones that say they are one hundred percent natural. Juices contain additives and added sugars. Such additives are not good for one's health.

Combining the Diets

There is no need to choose between intermittent fasting and the keto diet to achieve weight loss goals. It is possible and beneficial to combine these diets to optimize the benefits they offer. Doing this will not only promote weight loss, but it also helps control appetite, improve digestion and detoxify the body along the way. It is possible to amplify all these benefits while attaining ketosis so that the body is converted into a fat-burning machine. For instance, with the 5:2 method of intermittent fasting, caloric intake should be restricted to five hundred calories twice a week with unrestricted consumption on the other days of the week. To combine this protocol with the keto diet, all that is needed is to make sure that the foods consumed on the fasting days are keto-friendly. This means an emphasis on foods that are naturally fatty while limiting carbohydrate intake. The fatty foods that the keto diet recommends will produce fuller feeling for longer and will automatically reduce appetite. Such a high-fat diet therefore makes it easier to fast. The keto diet regulates sugar levels and restricts the production of hunger-inducing hormones like ghrelin. Caloric restriction when combined with a reduction of appetite automatically promotes weight loss.

When fasting restricts food intake, the body will reach into its internal stores of fats to provide energy. This process is known as ketosis and fasting makes it easier to transition into and maintain ketosis. The keto diet does not prescribe fasting, but combining these two diets will speed up the results. In the midst of fasting, the body automatically reaches into its internal fat stores to generate energy once all the glycogen is exhausted. Once this happens, it is quite easy to lose weight.

It is rather easy to combine these diets. The first step is selecting a preferred method of intermittent fasting. With a fasting protocol in hand, the next step is to eat foods that are keto-friendly. Then one must stick to the fasting window, and when it is time to eat, they must eat foods prescribed by the keto diet. For instance, if the method of fasting they opt for restricts the eating window from noon until 8 pm, then the food they eat during their feeding period must be keto-friendly. A guide like the keto food list discussed in this chapter will help identify what to eat and what to avoid.

If energy levels stay constant while appetite decreases, then it means that the combined diet is working well. However, before combining both of these diets, it is a good idea to start with intermittent fasting and then slowly incorporate the protocols of the ketogenic diet into the fold. There is value to observing the body's reaction to the diet in order to make the best adjustments for long-term success. Also, it is a good idea to always consult a doctor before deciding to start following any new diet or weight-loss program.

Chapter Eight:

What Works Best?

Effects of Intermittent Fasting on Women

It is essential to follow the protocols of intermittent fasting carefully; this is especially true for women. Women's bodies are usually more sensitive to any signals of starvation. Their bodies naturally misinterpret undereating as starvation, and this confusion leads to an increase in the production of the hunger hormones ghrelin and leptin. The presence of these hormones causes hunger pangs, even when the body does not need any extra nourishment. Whenever a woman's body senses that it is heading toward famine, regardless of whether it is intentional or not, it tends to secrete more of these hormones. These two hormones regulate hunger, and they give the body the signal that it is time to eat. So, whenever there is an increase in these hormones, it naturally creates a desire to eat.

Also, men's bodies function differently from women's. When a woman's body perceives that there is a shortage of nourishment (which might or might not be self-imposed), her body starts to shut down the reproductive system. The body does not have any desire to procreate and feels that there is not sufficient nourishment to sustain itself, let alone another being. This is the body's natural defense mechanism, and it kicks in when one does not carefully follow the protocols of intermittent fasting.

In the mammalian world, all mammals except human females are capable of terminating a pregnancy if the external factors are not favorable. Instead of being able to do this, a woman's body can shield itself from a potential pregnancy. A common side effect of intermittent fasting when it is not implemented correctly is that it can cause hormonal imbalances. Such imbalances can impact a woman's ability to conceive, the timing of her menstrual cycle, and other processes regulated by hormones. Despite these cautions, it is safe for women to intermittent fast (except when pregnant); they should be mindful and self-aware, performing frequent self-checks with regard to their physical condition and how they feel.

Who is Intermittent Fasting Ideal For?

Who can fast?
Healthy adults:

It is good for healthy adults to fast from time to time. It helps in cleansing the system. There is no reason why a healthy adult should not fast, except of course for pregnant women.

Children:

Children up to the age of eighteen do not need to fast. Although most children these days do not need to eat as frequently as they do, this does not mean they need to engage in extended periods of fasting. Fasting once in a while for short periods will not do them any harm.

Children need nutrition while growing up, but this does not mean that they should be overeating. If an obese child is under eighteen years of age, it is advisable to consult with a doctor before getting the child started on any form of diet, especially one that involves fasting for prolonged periods. As soon as the child starts eating healthily, there is no need for the child to fast any longer, unless of course there is a conscious effort to continue.

Type-2 diabetes:

Fasting has been used to reverse the effects of type-2 diabetes for a long time. There is a lot of research that backs the use of intermittent fasting as a tool to fight diabetes. Given the seriousness of the disease, those with type-2 diabetes should only begin a fasting regimen after consulting with a doctor.

Who must not fast?
Pregnant women:

Fasting's effect on an unborn fetus has not been thoroughly documented. However, it is believed that when a woman fasts while nursing, the milk produced is not as nutritious as it is supposed to be. There might be no difference in the amount of milk produced, however, the nutrient content in it is considered less. With the limited information currently available, caution is advised to ensure the safety of both mother and child.

Individuals with medical conditions:

Health issues related to the liver or kidneys normally exclude someone from fasting. Other conditions that may pose undue risk during fasting include: suffering from bouts of weakness, malnourishment, anemia, frailness, exhaustion. A person with any of these conditions should never begin fasting without the approval of a trusted doctor. Likewise, it is necessary to consult a doctor before fasting with any pre-existing medical conditions. Dependence on any medication, a weak immune system, high blood pressure, or poor circulation are also reasons to consult a doctor first. It is possible to fast comfortably while having a lot of pre-existing medical conditions, however, some conditions forbid certain individuals from fasting. If a person is on any medication, then the requirements of nutrition will vary. In any situation of doubt or uncertainty, it is always wise to consult a physician first.

Eating disorders:

Anyone with an eating disorder such as anorexia or bulimia must not fast. Fasting may not be advantageous to those with body dysmorphia.

After surgery:

In the aftermath of any major surgery, or recovery from any major illness, one must follow the doctor's treatment/recovery plan over any recommendation provided with respect to fasting.

Seamless Integration

Intermittent fasting is one of the most effective wellness strategies available these days. A rather enticing aspect of this varied eating plan is that it always provides the option of customization. One can schedule their eating and fasting periods based on convenience. As long as one stays mindful of what he or she eats during the eating window, then they should not have to worry about anything. But knowing about intermittent fasting and putting it into practice are two different things. Below are a couple of different tips that will undoubtedly come in handy when implementing this nutritional strategy.

Whenever a hunger pang is about to strike, it helps to take a couple of deep breaths and have a glass of water. The hunger pang should pass in less than fifteen minutes. If it does not ease up, a cup of green tea, herbal tea, or even black coffee should help.

When breaking a fast, gorging on food immediately is not the best way to transition from fasting to feasting. It is important to avoid greedily ingesting as much food as possible. Instead, it will help to take a couple of minutes and let the deep hunger pass before one starts eating more heavily. There is no rush. Eating slowly will provide an occasion to enjoy food all the more, since fasting has a way of piquing the senses of taste and smell. Eating less frequently also inspires gratitude. It is best to turn the TV off while eating, keep the phone away and avoid distractions. Mindless eating will rob you of eating's natural joy; on the other hand, mindful eating can help make the meal a celebration of life. There is a virtue in enjoying food and indulging the senses in the experience. Moderation is also of value. It might be necessary to develop a habit of resisting the urge to compensate for the fasting period by filling up with food. Such exuberance will not prove beneficial in the long run.

It is ideal to start the meal by having foods that are full of nutrients. So the goal is to have a plate full of food rich in proteins, natural fats, and fiber, instead of carbs and sugars. Protein and fiber will help produce a full feeling for longer and will help reduce caloric consumption as well. Nutrition must be the priority and not the quantity of food consumed. If the desire for a bowl of ice cream springs up, it must come after a full serving of nutritious food.

A colorful and varied plate should ensure adequate intake of micronutrients. Still, there can be additional health benefits to continuing with a regular supplement, and the great gains of intermittent fasting might even accelerate with the introduction of the right supplement or cocktail of supplements. Consensus opinion agrees that taking supplements while fasting does not hurt. There are practical considerations to keep in mind, like the fact that supplements can upset an empty stomach. Plenty of medical experts still doubt whether supplements even make a difference. But for those who deem them worthwhile, Dave Asprey, founder of Bulletproof Coffee, recommends a "biohacker" approach: take a supplement and see if there is a noticeable difference, either positive or negative.[17] Specific supplements that are popular within intermittent fasting circles include BCAAs, branched-chain amino acids, which bolster lean muscle mass, ensuring that there is no loss

---

[17] Asprey, D. (2019). Can You Take Supplements While Fasting? What You Need to Know. Retrieved from https://blog.bulletproof.com/supplements-while-fasting/

during fasting, exogenous ketones[18] to maximize energy from fat burning, and a basic multivitamin to avoid any blind-spot deficiencies.

Staying as busy as possible with little idle time will help in enduring fasting periods. If there is always work to demand attention, there will not be any spare time to think about hunger or dream about the next meal. A focus on food will result in feelings of hunger.

Overindulging during the initial couple of days of intermittent fasting is likely. When this happens, it is not a reason for panic or worry. It is just the body's survival instinct kicking in due to the absence of food. That survival instinct is hardwired into the brain, and it will take a week or two to recondition the body.

It is possible to maintain blood sugar levels throughout the day by having high-quality carbohydrates like vegetables and fruits along with a lot of protein and naturally fatty food during the eating window. It will also help the body to optimize its ability to burn stored fat.

With respect to sleep, adjusting the eating window to enable some time for digestion before lying down is beneficial. There may also be times when sleep is hindered by hunger pangs. Those instances will require some grit and determination. The feeling will come and go. But lack of sleep happens to be one of the most significant obstructions to losing weight, so it is important to get a good quality sleep at night. For optimal functioning of your body and brain, approximately eight hours of undisturbed sleep nightly is ideal.

---

[18] Axe, J. (2018, Dec. 6). The Intermittent Fasting Secret that No One is Talking About. Retrieved from https://store.draxe.com/blogs/all/intermittent-fasting-secret

Chapter Nine:

Fasting and Exercising

E ver since weights were introduced in gyms, the debate about whether it is better or worse to exercise on an empty stomach has been ongoing. This is a hotly debated topic, and the opinions offered differ frequently.

The body produces insulin via the pancreas upon ingestion of food, and that insulin helps the body utilize food's nutrient content. Insulin removes blood sugar from the blood and drives it to fat cells, muscles, and liver for future use. The problem usually lies in overeating, and often as a result, one's body may become less sensitive to insulin. Lower insulin sensitivity brings with it a host of other health issues, including an inability to lose body fat and a higher risk for cardiovascular disease and cancer. Eating less frequently, as is the case when one fasts intermittently, minimizes the body's production of insulin and, as such, lowers one's risk of becoming less and less sensitive to it over time. The less insulin the body needs to produce, the more vulnerable it becomes to it, which helps burn body fat and lower the risk of diabetes and cardiovascular disease.

Exercising on an empty stomach also helps the body concoct more HGH, which is essential for increasing muscle mass, stronger bones, fat burning, longevity, and improved physical functioning. Some studies have shown that a man's HGH production skyrockets by an astounding two thousand percent and a woman's by thirteen hundred percent when they fast for over twenty-four hours. Those gains come completely from not eating for twenty-four hours. Furthermore, those studies also showed that as soon as the fast is ended, HGH production plummets back down to normal. This is another reason to fast regularly and intermittently.

For men, it's virtually impossible to talk about muscle-building hormones without touching on the big T – testosterone. Testosterone is another powerful hormone that is responsible for muscle building, fat burning, higher energy levels, elevated libido and efficiently fighting off depression and heart problems. While intermittent fasting alone is not enough to significantly increase T levels, exercising on an empty stomach certainly can be.

If high-intensity compound exercises, i.e. those that involve a large number of muscles and muscle groups, can lead to a significant spike in testosterone levels, what more effective way to achieve this than to perform them while fasting intermittently? Studies have shown that working out this way under a state of fasting is one of the best ways to increase lean muscle mass and improve sensitivity to insulin. This happens due to hormonal responses and the body's ability to absorb more calories after each workout. It goes without saying that training while fasting intermittently significantly increases the likelihood that fat, protein and carbohydrate calories go to their respective destinations and minimizes the chances of them being stored as body fat.

Even if becoming more muscular is not the goal, exercising while fasting intermittently has other benefits to offer. Exercising on an empty stomach is especially useful for burning body fat and improving the ability to burn it at higher exercise intensity levels. For endurance athletes, intermittent fasting workouts can help improve the body's efficiency in storing glycogen. In layman's terms, periodically exercising with significantly depleted energy stores can help the body become even more efficient at using its energy stores.

Occasionally training on an empty stomach can help significantly improve the quality of non-fasting workouts later on. The bottom line is that when the body and its systems have become used to exertion without food, the capacity for exertion increases with a relatively full tank. Some researchers have demonstrated that fasted exercise sessions can dramatically increase endurance athletes' capacity to take in and utilize oxygen while exercising, which is an excellent way to evaluate their fitness level. In short, exercising on an empty stomach trains the body to perform more efficiently and effectively.

Yes, exercising on an empty stomach will help in optimizing the body's performance, leading to the oxidization of fat. However, if the goal is bulking up and performing high-intensity workouts, then the body does need some extra fuel.

To help fuel workouts, especially the first few after beginning intermittent fasting, one useful strategy is to drink more than just water. Pure green tea, pure black coffee, caffeine pills, creatine or just about any performance-enhancing supplements that are practically calorie-free can help. Caffeine is remarkable for its capability to boost endurance.

When working out intensely, breaking the fast in a purposeful way at any time of the day can help maximize training. Many athletes intentionally schedule their workouts in such a way that their first meal is right after working out. This is because anything they eat within the so-called post-exercise golden window (within 3 hours of working out), has very little chance of being stored as body fat. This will maximize the fat-loss benefits of exercising on an empty stomach.

If the normal routine is to exercise in the morning and have the first meal at noon, there is no need to worry. The spike in HGH production from working out on an empty stomach should be more than enough to prevent muscle loss (also known as muscle catabolism) during the day.

Humans are creatures of habit, and the human habit of eating is one of the most ingrained habits in our DNA. As such, eating less frequently may be a very challenging task to accomplish at first, especially if eating habits are ingrained rigidly. That is no cause for worry, though. All habits take time to break and replace. It has been said that habits, on average, take twenty-one straight days of practice before becoming new habits.

Conclusion

All the information provided in this book was expressed to help you understand what intermittent fasting is all about. Fasting, especially for prolonged periods, offers different benefits like improving one's overall metabolism, functioning of the body, and brain power. Intermittent fasting is based on two primary rules. The first rule is that you are free to eat only during the eating window, and the second rule is that you must opt for healthy and wholesome foods. During the fasting period, you need to ensure that your body is thoroughly hydrated. Intermittent fasting is a varied diet, and there are different protocols to intermittent fasting.

Depending on the goals you have set for yourself and the lifestyle you lead, you must opt for a method that best suits your needs and requirements. Selecting the right method can be a process of trial and error, so you might need to try a couple of methods before you find one that is ideal for you. Intermittent fasting doesn't induce any drastic changes that you must be worried about. It will just make you more mindful of what and when you are eating.

Please consult a doctor or medical practitioner before you start this diet. Apart from that, you can follow all the different steps and tips given in this book to kickstart autophagy. Also, if you want to speed up the process of weight loss, then you can always combine intermittent fasting with the keto diet.

It is my belief that YOU can easily attain your weight loss and fitness goals while improving your overall health by following this diet!

Now that you are armed with all the information you need, the next step is to get started as soon as you possibly can!

Thank you kindly – I wish you all the best!

Please click here to give "Intermittent Fasting" a review on Amazon!

Resources

Alirezaei, M., Kemball, C.C., Flynn, C.T., Wood, M.R., Whitton, J.L., & Kiosses, W.B. (2010). Short-term fasting induces profound neuronal autophagy. Retrieved from https://www.ncbi.nlm.nih.gov/pmc/articles/PMC3106288/

Asprey, D. (2019). Can You Take Supplements While Fasting? What You Need to Know. Retrieved from https://blog.bulletproof.com/supplements-while-fasting/

Axe, J. (2018, Dec. 6). The Intermittent Fasting Secret that No One is Talking About. Retrieved from https://store.draxe.com/blogs/all/intermittent-fasting-secret

The Beginner's Guide to the 5:2 Diet. (2019). Retrieved from https://www.healthline.com/nutrition/the-5-2-diet-guide

Belluz, J. (2018). What I learned about weight loss from spending a day inside a metabolic chamber. Retrieved from https://www.vox.com/2018/9/4/17486110/metabolism-diet-fast-weight-loss.

The Benefits of Dry Fasting - Dr. Mindy Pelz | Reset your Health. (2019). Retrieved from https://drmindypelz.com/the-benefits-of-dry-fasting/

Berg, J., Tymoczko, J., & Stryer, L. (2019). Glucose Can Be Synthesized from Noncarbohydrate Precursors. Retrieved from https://www.ncbi.nlm.nih.gov/books/NBK22591/

The Disadvantages of Fasting. (2019). Retrieved from https://healthyeating.sfgate.com/disadvantages-fasting-5546.html

Fong, J. [Transcript of podcast.] Retrieved from https://idmprogram.com/wp-content/uploads/Episode-14-Science-Transcript.pdf.

Forget Juice Cleanses. Autophagy Is the Real Way to Detox Your Body. (2019). Retrieved from https://blog.bulletproof.com/autophagy-for-longevity-detoxification/

Gandhi Begins Fast of 21 Days. (1943, Feb. 12). Retrieved from https://trove.nla.gov.au/newspaper/article/25940968

Gelino, S. & Hansen, M. (2019). Autophagy - An Emerging Anti-Aging Mechanism. Retrieved from https://www.ncbi.nlm.nih.gov/pmc/articles/PMC3674854/

Gustin, A. (2019). 16/8 Intermittent Fasting: How To Do It & Get The Health Benefits. Retrieved from https://perfectketo.com/16-8-intermittent-fasting-ketosis/

Ho, K.Y., Veldhuis, J.D., Johnson, M.L., Furlanetto, R., Evans, W.S., Alberti, K.G., & Thorner, M.O. (1988). Fasting enhances growth hormone secretion and amplifies the complex rhythms of growth hormone secretion in man. Retrieved from https://www.ncbi.nlm.nih.gov/pubmed/3127426

How to Fast Safely: Considerations Before Starting a Fast. (2019). Retrieved from https://www.globalhealingcenter.com/natural-health/how-to-fast-safely-considerations-before-fasting/

Kerndt, P.R., Naughton, J.L., Driscoll, C.E., & Loxterkamp, D.A. (1982 Nov.). Fasting: the history, pathophysiology and

complications. Retrieved from
https://www.ncbi.nlm.nih.gov/pubmed/6758355

Levy, J. (2018, Apr. 9). Benefits of Authophagy, Plus How to Induce It. Retrieved from https://draxe.com/benefits-of-autophagy/

Liu, W., Ye, L., Huang, W., Guo, L., Xu, Z., & Wu, H. et al. (2016). Cellular & Molecular Biology Letters, 21(1). doi: 10.1186/s11658-016-0031-z

The Nobel Prize in Physiology or Medicine 2016. (2019). Retrieved from https://www.nobelprize.org/prizes/medicine/2016/press-release/

Olsen, N.A. (2019). One meal a day: Health benefits and risks. Retrieved from https://www.medicalnewstoday.com/articles/320125.php

Pompa, D. (2018, Sept. 11). Fasting and Thyroid Conditions: Is it Possible? Retrieved from https://drpompa.com/fasting-diet/fasting-thyroid-conditions/

Solomon, S. (2015, Aug. 2). Fasting and Thyroid. Retrieved from https://www.drsarasolomon.com/fasting-and-thyroid/

Staughton, J. (2019, Feb. 10). 5 Scientifically Proven Benefits of Liquid Diet. Retrieved from https://owl.purdue.edu/owl/research_and_citation/apa_style/apa_formatting_and_style_guide/reference_list_electronic_sources.html

Stossel, J. (2019). Forget the hype; breakfast isn't important. Retrieved from https://www.palmbeachdailynews.com/article/20190411/OPINION/190419494.

Tabor, V.H. (2018, Oct. 19). Intermittent fasting, your thyroid, and your immune system. Retrieved from https://medium.com/boosted/intermittent-fasting-your-thyroid-and-your-immune-system-ec8f5f02d997

What Can You Drink While Fasting Without Breaking the Fast - Siim Land. (2019). Retrieved from http://siimland.com/what-can-you-drink-while-fasting/

The 12 Important Benefits Of Autophagy. (2019). Retrieved from https://www.naomiwhittel.com/the-12-important-benefits-of-autophagy/